No one would expect to understand a disease without knowledge of its clinical findings and pathology, but a surprising number of doctors remain ignorant of another important aspect – the study of disease in relation to populations. Epidemiology has its own techniques of data collection and interpretation and its necessary jargon of technical terms, and in *Epidemiology for the Uninitiated* Professors Geoffrey Rose and David Barker guide the novice expertly through the theory and practical pitfalls. The second edition of this popular *BMJ* handbook has been revised to include further details of epidemiological methods and some of their more dramatic applications, such as the investigations on the Spanish cooking oil epidemic, and AIDS.

EPIDEMIOLOGY FOR THE UNINITIATED

Second edition

GEOFFREY ROSE, DM, DSC, FRCP, FFCM

*Professor of epidemiology, Department of Epidemiology,
London School of Hygiene and Tropical Medicine, London*

D J P BARKER, PHD, MD, FRCP, FFCM

*Professor of clinical epidemiology and director,
Medical Research Council Environmental Epidemiology Unit,
University of Southampton, Southampton General Hospital,
Southampton*

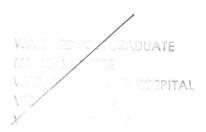

Articles from the *British Medical Journal*

Published by the British Medical Journal
Tavistock Square, London WC1H 9JR

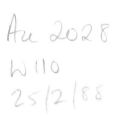

© British Medical Journal 1986

First published 1979
Third impression 1983
Second edition 1986
Second impression 1987

British Library Cataloguing in Publication Data

Rose, Geoffrey, *1926-*
 Epidemiology for the uninitiated.—2nd ed.
 1. Epidemiology
 I. Title   II. Barker, D J P   III. British
Medical Association
 614.4   RA651

ISBN 0-7279-0177-X

Printed in Great Britain by
Latimer Trend & Co Ltd, Plymouth

Preface

to the second edition

Few things are more dispiriting for a medical editor than having to reject a paper based on a good idea but with irremediable flaws in the methods used. All too often doctors set about research projects without having asked advice on the best way to compare populations or to carry out surveys.

The articles that make up this book were commissioned from Professor Geoffrey Rose and Professor David Barker, two of our leading epidemiologists, with the aim of helping future authors to avoid the most obvious traps. They have now been revised and brought up to date for this second edition. The information they contain will also help readers of medical journals to make more sense of the articles they contain—and to judge for themselves whether the conclusions are valid.

STEPHEN LOCK
Editor
British Medical Journal

Contents

What is epidemiology?

Epidemiology is the study of disease in relation to populations. Like the clinical findings and pathology, the epidemiology of a disease is an integral part of its basic description. The subject has its special techniques of data collection and interpretation, and its necessary jargon for technical terms. It will be the aim of this short book to provide for the uninitiated an ABC of the epidemiological approach, its terminology, and its methods. Our only assumption will be that readers already believe that epidemiological questions are worth answering. This introduction will indicate some of the distinctive characteristics of the epidemiological approach, especially those which differ from the familiar clinical descriptive methods.

All findings must relate to a defined population

Whereas clinical studies are carried out on patients, epidemiology, which seeks to relate disease to the population in which it occurs, requires study of both sick and healthy. If findings in the cases cannot be related to the defined population in which those cases arose, then it is not epidemiology.

This *population at risk* is a basic concept of epidemiology. In a study of accidents to patients in hospital it was noted that the largest number occurred among the elderly, and from this the authors concluded that "patients aged 60 and over are most prone to accidents." Another study, based on a survey of hang gliding accidents, recommended that flying should be banned between 11 am and 3 pm, because this was the time when 73% of the accidents occurred. Each of these studies based conclusions on the same logical error, namely, the *floating numerator*: the number of cases was not related to the appropriate "at risk" population. Had this been done, the conclusions might have been different. Differing *numbers* of accidents to patients and to hang gliders must reflect, at least in part, differing numbers at risk. Epidemiological conclusions (on risk) cannot be drawn from purely clinical data (on the frequency of sick people seen).

What is a population? Statisticians, demographers, and epidemiologists would answer differently. Epidemiologically it means a defined group, including both sick and healthy, about whose health some statement is to be made. In practice, it is unlikely that the whole of this *target population* can or needs to be examined, access being limited to some subset of it—the *study population*. Thus a chemical pathologist wishing to establish a range of normal values may investigate the employees of a local factory, hoping that they represent the generality of healthy people. The process of inference (generalisation) from study to target population is a matter for judgment, not statistics.

Even the study population will usually be larger than the investigation requires, and actual examination may be limited to a *study sample*. Thus the people examined are now at two removes from the group with which the study is ultimately concerned:

Target population→study population→study sample

The study sample is of interest only in so far as it shows what is happening in the population. Inference from sample to study population is rigorous and statistical, provided that the sample is representative. This requires (*a*) an unambiguous *definition* of who is eligible for the study population; (*b*) an enumeration or *census* of all its members; (*c*) a *sampling* process such that each member has a known (usually equal) probability of selection into the study sample. Probability sampling does not guarantee representativeness, but it does allow the limits of sampling error to be precisely calculated.

The definition of the study population begins with some basic characteristic which all its members have in common. This may be *geographical* ("all UK residents in 1985", or "all residents in a certain health district"); *occupational* ("all employees of a factory", "children attending a certain primary school", "all instrument and watchmakers and precision tool operators in England and

2

Wales"*); or *based on special care* ("a GP's list", "residents in an old people's home", "all persons coming to autopsy").

Within this broad definition appropriate restrictions may be specified—for example, in age range or sex.

Oriented to groups rather than individuals

Clinical observations determine decisions about individuals. Epidemiological observations determine decisions about groups, being the basis for preventive policy and health care planning.

This fundamental difference in the purpose of measurements implies different demands on the quality of data. An inquiry into the validity of death certificates as an indicator of the frequency of oesophageal cancer produced the following results:

Diagnosed by clinician	74
Confirmed by pathologist	53
Not confirmed by pathologist	21
First diagnosed post mortem	22

Inaccuracy was alarming at the level of individual patients. Nevertheless, the false positive errors balanced the false negatives, and so the clinicians' total (74 cases) was about the same as the pathologists' total (53 + 22 = 75 cases). Hence in this instance mortality statistics in the population seemed to be about right, despite the unreliability of any individual death certificate. In other instances there could be serious bias. Conversely, it may not be too serious clinically if "Doctor X" systematically records blood pressure 10 mm Hg higher than his colleagues, because his management policy is (one hopes) adjusted accordingly. But in a population study of the frequency of hypertension, choosing "Doctor X" as observer would be unfortunate.

Conclusions are based on comparisons

Clues to *aetiology* come from comparing disease rates in groups with differing levels of exposure—for example, increase in congenital defects after a rubella epidemic, excess lung cancer and pleural mesothelioma in those exposed to asbestos. Clues will be missed, or false clues created, if comparisons are biased by unequal

---

*A group reported to have excessive mortality from arthritis and anaemia, possibly due to potent treatments given because their work demands supple fingers.

ascertainment of cases or exposure levels. Of course, if everyone is equally exposed there will not be any clues—epidemiology thrives on heterogeneity. If everyone smoked 20 cigarettes daily the link with lung cancer would have been undetectable. Lung cancer would then have been considered a "genetic disease", because its distribution depended on susceptibility.

Identifying *high risk* and *priority groups* again rests on unbiased comparison of rates. From the *Decennial Occupational Supplement of the Registrar General of England and Wales* (1970–2) it appears that there are major differences between occupations in the proportion of men surviving to age 65:

Farmers (self employed)	82%
Professionals	77%
Skilled manual workers	69%
Labourers	63%
Armed forces	42%

These differences look important and challenging. Firstly, however, one must consider how far the comparison may have been biased in ascertainment of either the deaths or the populations at risk, or by selective influences on recruitment or retirement (especially important in the case of the armed forces).

Another task of epidemiology is *monitoring* or *surveillance* of time trends to show which diseases are increasing, which decreasing, and which changing in their distribution. This information is needed for the identification of both emerging problems and of the effectiveness of measures to control old ones. Unfortunately, standards of diagnosis and data recording may change, and conclusions from time trends call for particular wariness.

The data from which epidemiology seeks to draw conclusions are nearly always collected by more than one person, often from different countries. Rigorous *standardisation* and *quality control* of investigative methods demand major emphasis in epidemiology; and if an apparent difference in disease rates has emerged, the first question is always "Might the comparison be biased?"

What is a case? Dichotomy or continuum?

In clinical practice the definition of "a case" generally assumes that in any disease people are divided into two discrete classes—the affected and the unaffected. This assumption works well enough in the hospital ward, and at one time it was thought appropriate also for populations. Cholera, for instance, was identified only by an attack of profuse watery diarrhoea, often fatal; but we now know that infection may also be subclinical, or cause only mild diarrhoea. Similarly in non-infectious diseases today we recognise the importance of premalignant dysplasias, in situ carcinoma, mild hypertension, and presymptomatic airways obstruction in smokers. Increasingly it appears that disease in populations exists as a continuum of severity rather than as an all or none phenomenon. The rare exceptions are mainly genetic disorders with high penetrance, like achondroplasia; for most acquired diseases the real question in population studies is not "Has he got it?" but "How much of it has he got?"

In the first place quantitative results should always be reported quantitatively, as distributions of their relevant statistics—for example, mean and standard deviation. Arbitrary cut off points waste information and can prevent communication. In one study (table I) estimates of diabetes prevalence ranged from 7% to 32%, depending on which of various "standard" definitions was adopted.

5

TABLE I—*Bedford diabetes survey: effect on prevalence estimate of different criteria for glucose tolerance test results*

Criterion	Prevalence
≥ 120 mg/100 ml (6·7 mmol/l) @ 2 h	16%
≥ 140 mg/100 ml (7·8 mmol/l) @ 2 h	7%
≥ 180 mg/100 ml (10 mmol/l) @ peak	32%
≥ 120 mg/100 ml @ 2 h *and* > 180 mg/100 ml @ peak	11%

What is abnormal?

For practical reasons even quantitative results must often be divided into acceptable and unacceptable. In defining cut off points four approaches may be considered:

Statistical—"Normal" may be defined as within two standard deviations of the age specific mean, following conventional laboratory practice. This is acceptable as a simple guide to the limits of what is common; but it must not be given any other significance, for it fixes the frequency of "abnormal" values of every variable at around 5% in every age and population. More importantly, what is common is not necessarily good.

Clinical—Clinical significance may be defined as the level of a variable above which symptoms and complications become more frequent. This level may be hard to identify. Anaemia is traditionally associated with tiredness, and so a woman attending her doctor with this complaint is likely to have a blood count. In this way anaemia is more likely to be discovered in tired than in other patients, and the association becomes a self fulfilling prophecy. In a population survey employing uniform standards of ascertainment it was impossible to prove any overall excess of symptoms among those with haemoglobin concentrations down to 8 g/dl.

Prognostic—In a man of 50 a systolic pressure of 150 mm Hg is common (that is, "statistically normal"), and it is clinically normal, in the sense of being symptomless; but his risk of fatal heart attack is about twice that of his contemporary with a low blood pressure. In fact, the prognostically ideal blood pressure seems to be "as low as possible", and in this sense the concept of "a case of hypertension" becomes inappropriate.

Sometimes, as with glucose tolerance, there may be a threshold value below which level and prognosis are unrelated. "Prognostically abnormal" is then definable by this level. In other instances, as with body weight, the relation to prognosis is U shaped: the highest mortality rates occur at the two extremes of the distribution, creating categories both "abnormally high" and "abnormally low".

Operational—The research worker may be content to describe his distributions, but for the man of action dichotomy is unavoidable: however arbitrary may be the definitions of hypertension or diabetes, a decision has to be taken that at some level patients should be treated. This operational definition will take into account the clinical and prognostic definitions, but it may well differ from either: a person may be symptom free yet benefit by treatment, or, alternatively, he may have an increased risk which cannot be remedied. For screening, a case should be defined in relation to that level of disease above which action is better than inaction.

Each of these four approaches to case definition is suitable for a different purpose, so the investigator may need to define his purpose before he can define his cases.

Definitions and descriptions

A standard textbook of cardiology proposes these electrocardiographic criteria for left bundle branch block: "The duration of QRS *commonly* measures 0·12 to 0·16 seconds ... V5 or V6 exhibits a *large widened* R wave ..." (*our italics*). As a basis for epidemiological comparisons this is potentially disastrous, since each investigator could interpret the italicised words in his own way. By contrast, the epidemiological "Minnesota Code" defines it like this: "QRS duration $\geqslant$ 0·12 seconds in any one or more limb leads *and* R peak duration $\geqslant$ 0·06 seconds in any one or more of leads, I, II, aVL, V5, or V6; each criterion to be met in a majority of technically adequate beats." If different studies are to be compared, case definitions must be rigorously standardised and free of ambiguity. Conventional clinical descriptions do not meet this requirement.

It is also essential to define and standardise the methods of measuring the chosen criteria. An important feature in diagnosing rheumatoid arthritis, for example, is early morning stiffness of the fingers; but two interviewers may emerge with different prevalence estimates if one takes an ordinary clinical history while the other uses a standard questionnaire. Cases in a survey are defined not by theoretical criteria, but in terms of response to specific investigative techniques. These, too, need to be defined, standardised, and adequately reported. As a result epidemiological case definitions are narrower and more rigid than clinical ones. This loss of flexibility has to be accepted as the price of standardisation.

Defining the source of cases

Cases derived from different sources cannot necessarily be compared, even if an identical case definition has been used. Table II shows the results from a large screening survey using rigorously standardised reporting: identical electrocardiographic findings are seen to carry a very different prognosis according to whether they were first found at screening, or arose in men already under

TABLE II—*Prognosis of ECG findings at screening of 18 403 middle aged men, according to whether they were already under medical care*

	Five year CHD mortality (%)	
	Not under care	Under care
Prominent Q-wave	3·4	6·3
S-T segment depression	3·2	13·3
Normal ECG	*1·0*	*5·1*

medical care. Before statements are made about disease and its outcome it is essential to define the source of the cases and the selective processes affecting entry to the study. Failure to do so, which is one of the commonest faults in epidemiological papers, prevents generalisation of the conclusions and comparison with other studies.

Rates

Rates are the hallmark of epidemiology, for they form the basis of comparisons between population groups. "Floating numerators" are anathema, for they cannot be interpreted.

A choice of denominators

Most rates take the form:

$$\frac{\text{Frequency of observed state or event}}{\text{Total number in whom this state or event } might \text{ occur}}$$

The denominator consists of all those, and only those, who might appear in the numerator. Such a rate expresses the proportion of the population that is affected, and also the average risk of being affected for any particular member of it. In a survey unexamined individuals are clearly not at risk of being recognised as cases, and rates are usually based on a denominator of respondents. This introduces an error, because rates in non-respondents are likely to be different.

In rates for populations and in follow up studies the denominator may be constantly changing owing to births, deaths, migrations, and other losses. The denominator may then be taken as the average of the initial and final numbers. If losses occur irregularly during the study it is better to use the exact number of *person years at risk*. In this way, the results in the table identified an association—still unexplained—between coronary heart disease risk and exposure to carbon disulphide. The same approach is useful in dealing with dropouts in clinical trials and follow up studies.

The figure shows an apparently alarming increase in the propor-

Death rates (age adjusted) from coronary heart disease in a viscose rayon factory

Occupational group	Man years at risk	CHD mortality per 1000 man years
Viscose spinners	6087	9·0
Others	4970	3·7

tion of anaesthetic deaths due to accidents, but the trend was due entirely to a large decline in the non-accidental deaths. The actual number of accidental deaths had not increased at all. This shows the danger of relating cases not to the real "at risk" population, but to the "total of patients" (operations, hospital admissions, necropsies, GP consultations). Where the population is unknown there may, however, be no alternative.

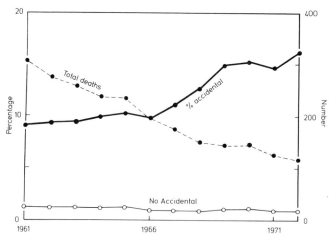

Deaths under or connected with anaesthesia: total, and number and percentage attributable to accidents (England and Wales, moving averages).

Measures of disease frequency

Measures of disease frequency may express *morbidity*, which is the frequency of illness and disability, or *mortality*, the frequency of death. They may be classed also as measures of *prevalence* (static) or *incidence* (kinetic).

Prevalence rate

The prevalence rate is *the proportion of a defined group having a condition at one point in time*. The prevalence of persistent phlegm production in middle aged men in Britain has been estimated at about 10%, the condition being defined by response to a standard questionnaire. Prevalence is an appropriate measure only in such relatively stable conditions, and it is unsuitable for acute conditions.

Even in a chronic disease the manifestations are often intermittent. In consequence, a "point" prevalence rate, based on a single examination at one point in time, tends to underestimate the condition's total frequency. If repeated assessments of the same individuals are possible, a better measure is the *period prevalence rate*, defined as *the proportion of a defined group having a condition at any time within a stated period*. In one study the point prevalence rate of angina in middle aged working men was estimated at 4%. The same interview technique applied annually in the same men yielded a five year period prevalence rate of 10%: many men lost not only their symptoms but also, apparently, their memory of them. In this way many chronic conditions are probably much commoner than is supposed.

SOME SPECIAL RATES

Birth rate	$\dfrac{\text{Number of live births}}{\text{Mid-year population}}$
Fertility rate	$\dfrac{\text{Number of live births}}{\text{Number of women aged 15–44 years}}$
Infant mortality rate	$\dfrac{\text{Number of infant } (<1 \text{ year}) \text{ deaths}}{\text{Number of live births}}$
Stillbirth rate	$\dfrac{\text{Number of intrauterine deaths after 28 weeks}}{\text{Total births}}$
Perinatal mortality rate	$\dfrac{\text{Number of stillbirths} + \text{deaths in 1st week of life}}{\text{Total births}}$

NB These rates are usually related to one year.

Incidence rate

The incidence rate is the *proportion of a defined group developing a condition within a stated period*. In clinical use incidence often refers to a *frequency*—that is, a number of cases. Epidemiologically it is a *proportion*—that is, a number of cases related to a defined population and a stated period of time.

Incidence measures the rate of occurrence of new cases. At least two examinations are implied. At the first, cases already having the condition are excluded from further analysis. They cannot contribute to the numerator, which consists of new cases; and so they also cannot appear in the denominator, which consists only of persons at risk of qualifying for the numerator. Further, only those new cases who are included in the "at risk" population must be counted. Thus a general practitioner using his practice list to define the population must exclude from the study patients who are only visitors.

Incidence studies are more complex than prevalence studies and, because incidence rates tend to be low, they require large populations.

Incidence rate (spells)

Sometimes the same pathological event happens more than once to the same individual. For a conventional incidence rate only the first event qualifies, but in the absence of some form of record linkage it may be impossible to identify multiple events affecting one individual. This happens in the Hospital Inpatient Inquiry, which is an annually published analysis of hospital cases in England and Wales: the numerator is the total number of discharges (and deaths) for a particular disease, and there is no way of telling how many patients are concerned. The same often holds for general practice consultation rates, occupational sickness absence rates, and venereal disease diagnosis rates. Incidence must then be related to episodes, not persons; thus the "incidence rate (spells)" is *the total number of episodes in a stated period related to the "at risk" population*.

Such rates need to be interpreted with caution. For example, gonorrhoea notification rates have increased dramatically; but no one knows to what extent this is due to more people getting infected or to the same people getting infected more often.

Prevalence, incidence, and outcome

Each new (incidence) case enters the prevalence pool and remains there until either recovery or death:

$$Incidence \rightarrow Prevalence \begin{cases} \rightarrow Recovery \\ \rightarrow Death \end{cases}$$

If recovery and death rates are low, then chronicity is high and even a low incidence rate will produce a high prevalence:

$$Prevalence = incidence \times average\ duration$$

Surgical advances in the treatment of spina bifida dramatically reduced the mortality rate, but in the absence of true recovery this greatly increased the prevalence of serious disability. Prevalence rates cannot therefore be taken as simple reflections of incidence rates, because they depend also on outcome and the availability of effective treatment. An adequate description of disease in a population is kinetic as well as static.

Crude and specific rates

A crude rate is one which relates to results for the study population taken as a whole, without subdivision or refinement. To state that the crude mortality rate in England and Wales in 1983 was 11·6 per 1000 per year is medically uninformative: it can be used in demographic estimates of population size, but it tells us little about the health of the nation. The simplest refinement is a "cause specific" rate, which permits comparisons between different causes within the same population.

If comparisons are to be made between populations, it may be helpful to break results down further—for example, by age and sex. It is frustrating if results are given for 35–44 years in one report, 30–49 in another, and 31–40 in another. Where feasible, decade classes should therefore be 5–14, 15–24, and so on, and quinquennia should be 5–9, 10–14, and so on. Overlapping classes (5–10, 10–15) should be avoided.

Observer variation

Observational data derived from whole populations are crude and often inaccurate, and comparisons when different observers are used are particularly fraught with danger. The epidemiologist has to apply intellectual rigour to interpreting weak data, and his motto could well be "dirty hands, but a clean mind" (*manus sordidae, mens pura*). Observer variation is also important in clinical practice, but the demands of epidemiology have given a special fillip to its study. It is primarily the basis for assessing the quality of the data, and then for improving that quality.

Collecting the information

Every epidemiological study should include for its main measurements some check of their repeatability (also known, less satisfactorily, as "precision" and "reliability"). This is best built into the main study—either a sample of subjects undergoing a second examination, or a sample of x ray films, blood samples, and so on being tested in duplicate. Even a small sample is valuable, provided that (1) it is representative, and (2) the duplicate tests are genuinely independent, the observer being unable to identify the pairs. If testing is done "off line" (perhaps as part of a pilot study), then particular care is needed to ensure that subjects, observers, and operating conditions are all adequately representative of the main study. It is much easier to test repeatability when the data can be transported and stored—for example, deep frozen plasma samples, histological sections, and all kinds of tracings and photographs. Nevertheless, such tests may exclude an important source of observer variation—namely, the techniques of obtaining samples and records.

Identifying the components of error

Independent replicate measurements in the same subjects are usually found to vary more than one's gloomiest expectations. To interpret the results, and to seek remedies, it is helpful to dissect the total variability into its four components:

Within observer variation—Discovering one's own inconsistency can be traumatic; it highlights a lack of clear criteria of measurement and interpretation, particularly in dealing with the grey area between "normal" and "abnormal". It is largely *random*—that is, unpredictable in direction.

Between observer variation—This includes the first component (the instability of individual observers), but adds to it an extra and *systematic* component due to individual differences in technique and criteria. Unfortunately, this may be large in relation to the real difference between the groups which it was hoped to identify.

It may be possible to avoid the problem altogether, either by using a single observer or, if data are transportable, by forwarding them all for central examination. Alternatively, the bias within one survey may be neutralised by random allocation of subjects to observers. Each observer should also be identified by a code number on the survey record; analysis of results by observer will then identify major problems, and perhaps permit some statistical correction for the bias.

Random subject variation—When measured repeatedly in the same subject, physiological variables like blood pressure tend to show an approximately normal distribution around the subject's mean. Nevertheless, surveys usually have to make do with a single measurement, and the error will not be noticed unless the extent of subject variation has been studied.

Random subject variation has some important implications for screening and also in clinical practice, when subjects with extreme initial values are recalled. Thanks to a statistical quirk this group then appears to improve, for its members include some whose mean value is normal but who by chance were above this value at first examination: on average, their follow up values necessarily tend to fall (*regression to the mean*). The size of this effect depends on the amount of random subject variation. Misinterpretation can be avoided by repeated examinations to establish an adequate baseline, or else (in an intervention study) by including a control group.

Biased (systematic) subject variation—Blood pressure is much influenced by the temperature of the examination room, as well as by less readily standardised emotional factors. Afternoon surveys of patients with diabetes find a much higher prevalence than morning surveys; and possibly the standard bronchitis questionnaire elicits more positive responses in winter than in summer. Thus conditions and timing of an investigation may have a major effect on an individual's true state and on his responses. Such sources of biases are often unrecognised, and even when recognised they may be hard to control. Studies should therefore be designed so that they will not distort the crucial comparisons.

Implications of variability

The practical consequences of variability depend less on whether the error is due to observer or subject than on whether it is random or biased.

Random error

(1) Individuals are apt to be misassessed or misclassified. This is serious in clinical practice and in screening, both of which are concerned with the correct management of individuals; but it is not in itself serious in epidemiology, which is mainly concerned with correct decisions about groups.

(2) The mean value for a group is estimated with less certainty (that is, its standard error is increased), but fortunately this uncertainty may be reduced *to any required extent* simply by increasing the sample size, or by replicating measurements in individuals. The strength of epidemiology (and one that clinicians may be inclined to question) is its ability to tolerate crude and inaccurate measuring techniques, provided that sample size and study design are adequate.

(3) An important exception to epidemiology's ability to tolerate random individual errors is in the search for within subject associations, such as genetic and other risk factors. Random error

in the measurements will necessarily tend to cloud true associations and to underestimate true correlations: if crude methods can demonstrate a significant correlation, one may be reasonably sure that its real magnitude is greater than appears.

(4) The size of all these errors from random variation can be estimated, provided that the investigator included an inquiry into measurement variability.

All error in measurements is undesirable; but, provided its size is known, random error can generally be tolerated. It is "clean dirt".

Biased error

(1) By definition this biases conclusions about groups (means or rates) and distorts comparisons. Epidemiologically, this is fatal.

(2) Its effects are in no way reduced by an increase in sample size, a large study that is biased being no better than a small one. (Indeed, it is worse, because it is more likely to be believed.)

(3) It is often unrecognised or hard to quantify. Efforts to compensate for it in the analysis must be viewed with suspicion.

Biased error strikes at the roots of comparisons. It is "dirty dirt", and in epidemiology it cannot be tolerated.

Repeatability and validity

An ideal survey technique is repeatable (it gives the same answer when the subject is re-examined) and also valid (it measures what it purports to measure). Poor repeatability implies poor validity, because only one answer can be the right one. But a consistent answer may also be wrong: a laboratory test may yield persistently false positive results, or a highly repeatable psychiatric questionnaire may be an insensitive measure of, for example, "stress". To assess how much weight to attach to epidemiological results calls for numerical estimates of both their repeatability and their validity.

Repeatability

The principles of repeatability testing were described in the last chapter. Results for numerical variables such as blood pressure may be expressed as the *standard deviation* of replicate measurements or as the *coefficient of variation* (standard deviation ÷ mean). Separate estimates may be given for within and between observers, or for variability between measurements made consecutively and those made on separate occasions.

For qualitative attributes, such as clinical symptoms and signs, the results are first set out as a contingency table:

		Observer 1	
		Positive	Negative
Observer 2	Positive	a	b
	Negative	c	d

The overall level of agreement could be represented by the proportion of the total falling in cells a and d. This measure unfortunately turns out to depend more on the prevalence of the condition than on the repeatability of the method. This is because in practice it is easy to agree on a straightforward negative; disagreements depend on the prevalence of the difficult borderline cases. *Repeatability (for the individual subject)* is usually therefore defined as:

$$\frac{\text{Number of agreed positive}}{\text{Number positive to either observer}} = \frac{a}{a+b+c}$$

This measure is largely independent of prevalence. It states the probability, given one positive test, of the second also being positive.

Epidemiological conclusions are more concerned with groups than individuals, and the above measure is less important than an estimate of *observer* or *test bias*:

$$\frac{\text{Number positive to observer 1}}{\text{Number positive to observer 2}} = \frac{a+c}{a+b}$$

Note that agreed positives are necessarily fewer than the positives for a single observer. *The apparent frequency of any condition is inversely proportional to the number of investigators (or investigations) required to establish its presence.*

Measuring validity

A sphygmomanometer's validity can be measured by comparing its readings with intra-arterial pressures, and the validity of a mammographic diagnosis of breast cancer can be tested (if the woman agrees) by biopsy. More often, however, there is no sure reference standard. The validity of a questionnaire for diagnosing angina cannot be fully known: the best clinical opinion is subject to observer variation, and even coronary arteriograms may be normal in true cases or abnormal in symptomless people. The pathologist can describe post mortem structural changes, but these may say little of the patient's symptoms or functional state. Measurements of disease in life, whether clinical or epidemiological, are often incapable of full validation.

In practice, therefore, validity may have to be assessed indirectly. In epidemiology two approaches are available. A test which has been simplified and standardised to make it suitable for use in surveys may then be compared with the best conventional clinical assessment. A self administered psychiatric questionnaire, for instance, may be compared with the majority opinion of a psychiatric panel. Alternatively, a test may be validated by its ability to predict an abnormal glucose tolerance test, or of a questionnaire to predict future illness. Validation, especially by predictive ability, tends to be more difficult and to require much larger numbers than the testing of repeatability.

Analysing validity

The same subjects are classified as positive or negative, first by the survey and secondly by the reference test, and the findings can then be expressed in a contingency table:

Survey test	Reference test		Totals
	Positive	Negative	
Positive	True positives, correctly identified = (a)	False positives = (b)	Total test positives = (a + b)
Negative	False negatives, = (c)	True negatives, correctly identified = (d)	Total test negatives = (c = d)
Totals	Total true positives = (a + c)	Total true negatives = (b + d)	Grand total = (a + b + c + d)

From this table four important statistics can be derived.

Sensitivity—A sensitive test detects a high proportion of the true cases, and this quality is measured here by $a/a + c$.

Specificity—A specific test has few false positives, and this quality is measured by $d/b + d$.

Systematic error—For epidemiological rates it is particularly important for the test to give the right total count of cases. This is measured by the ratio of the total numbers positive to the survey and the reference tests, or $(a + b)/(a + c)$.

Predictive value—This is the proportion of test positives that are truly positive. It is important in screening, and will be discussed later (p 44).

It should be noted that both systematic error and predictive value must depend on the relative frequency of true positives and true negatives in the particular study group (that is, on prevalence of abnormality).

Sensitive or specific? A matter of choice

If diagnostic criteria are stringent there will be few false positives but the test will be insensitive. Conversely, if criteria are relaxed there will be fewer false negatives but the test will be less specific. In a recent survey of breast cancer alternative diagnostic criteria were compared in relation to a reference test (positive biopsy). Clinical palpation by a doctor yielded fewest false positives (93% specificity), but missed half the cases (50% sensitivity). Criteria for "a case" were then relaxed to include all the positives identified by doctor's palpation, nurse's palpation, or x ray mammography: few cases were now missed (94% sensitivity), but specificity fell to 86%.

By choosing the right test and cut off points it may be possible to get the balance of sensitivity and specificity that is best for the particular study. In a survey to establish prevalence this might be when false positives balance false negatives. In a study to compare rates in different populations the absolute rates are less important, the primary concern being to avoid systematic bias: a specific test is likely to be preferred, even at the price of some loss of sensitivity.

Planning a survey

Medical planning requires information on the extent and distribution of health problems. These are often not available, especially at a local level. A geriatrician asks about the extent of unmet need among district residents. An inner city psychiatrist wants to back his request for more facilities by some evidence of high local morbidity. A physician needs to know how much hypertension would be uncovered if blood pressures were measured in non-medical clinics. A general practitioner wonders if there really is a local excess of bronchitis. A chemical pathologist wishes to establish a "range of normal". In some such ways almost any doctor may find himself needing to undertake a simple cross sectional survey. We will attempt to help him in this chapter and the next.

Early planning

Actual data collection begins only late; its success depends on careful preparation, often requiring many months.

Background reading

Library research may uncover unsuspected sources of published information (for instance, the Registrar General's mortality and cancer registry reports, the Hospital Inpatient Inquiry, the reports on morbidity in general practice). The Regional Hospital Activity Analysis may provide special tabulations on request. Similar surveys may have been done elsewhere. Even if the library does not yield the whole answer it often guides the planning.

Defining specific questions

The first and often the most difficult question is "Why am I doing this survey?" Many studies start with a general hope that something interesting will emerge, and they often end in frustration. The general interest has first to be translated into precisely formulated, written objectives. Every survey should be reasonably sure to give an adequate answer to at least one specific question. This initial planning requires some idea of the final analysis; and it may be useful at the outset to outline the key tables for the final report, and to consider the numbers of cases expected in their major cells.

Every study needs a primary purpose. It is easy to argue, "While we have the subjects there, let's also measure . . ."; but overloading, whether of investigators or subjects, must be avoided if it in any way threatens the primary purpose. Sometimes subsidiary objectives may be pursued in subsamples (every nth subject, or in a particular age group), or by recalling some subjects for a second examination: when their initial contact has been favourable, response to recall is usually good.

Choice of examination methods

The overriding need in an epidemiological survey is to examine a representative sample of adequate size in a standardised and sufficiently valid way. This determines the choice of examination methods and the points where these differ from those of clinical practice. Methods must be acceptable, and if possible non-invasive, or else cooperation suffers and the study group becomes unrepresentative. They must be relatively cheap and quick, or not enough subjects can be examined: with fixed resources the need for detail conflicts with the need for numbers. Most important of all, methods and observers must be capable of rigorous standardisation; even if this excludes the benefits of clinical judgment.

The price of these necessary characteristics of epidemiological methods may be a substantial loss of validity (sensitivity or specificity or both) and, in the interests of making fair comparisons between populations, conclusions about individuals in the study will be limited.

23

Sampling

Sample size

Most surveys and trials are smaller than the investigator would wish, lack of numbers often setting a limit to some desirable subgroup analysis. This is inevitable. What can be avoided is discovering only at the final analysis that numbers do not permit achievement even of the study's primary objective. To prevent this disappointment the purpose of the study has first to be formulated in precise statistical terms. If the aim is to estimate prevalence, then sample size will depend on the required accuracy of that esimate. (The table gives some examples.) Sampling error is proportionally greater for less common conditions; that is to say, to achieve the same level of confidence requires a larger sample if prevalence is low. Doubling the size of the study does not double its accuracy; in fact, it reduces the standard error by a factor of $\sqrt{2}$.

Techniques also exist for calculating sample sizes required for estimating, with specified precision, the mean value of a variable, or for identifying a given difference in prevalence or mean values between two populations. These techniques may be found in the textbooks or (better) by consulting a statistician; but either way the investigator must first know exactly what he wants to achieve.

95% confidence limits for various rates and sample sizes

Estimated prevalence (%)	95% confidence limits	
	n = 500	n = 1000
2	1·0–3·7	1·2–3·1
10	7·5–13·0	8·2–12·0
20	16·6–23·8	17·6–22·6

Sampling methods

Statistical inference is possible only if the sample is random, or effectively random; that is to say, if each individual in the study population has a known (usually identical) probability of selection. To achieve this a *census* or listing of the study population is first required. In a survey of adults in a hospital district the electoral register will probably serve. In an occupational group the payroll is invariably complete, and in a school there are class registers. In general practice there may be an age-sex register (although many are inaccurate); otherwise a *systematic sample* may be obtained by taking the notes of every nth patient, and this should be adequately representative.

In a *simple random sample* the listed subjects are numbered serially. Numbers within the appropriate range are then read off from a table of random numbers until enough subjects have been chosen.

It may be that the investigator wishes to choose a sample in which certain subgroups (particular ages, for instance, or high risk categories) are relatively overrepresented. To achieve this he may divide the study population into subgroups (*strata*) and then draw a separate random sample from each, while adjusting the various sample sizes to suit his requirements. This is a *stratified random sample*.

The study population may be large and widely scattered—for example, all the general practices in a city—but for the sake of convenience the investigator may wish to concentrate his survey in a few areas only. He can do this by drawing first a random sample of practices, and then, within these practices, drawing a random sample of individuals. This is *two stage sampling*. There is some loss in statistical efficiency, especially if at the first stage only a few units are selected. If the acceptable number of first stage units is very small then random selection is unsuitable, judgment serving better than chance.

Conduct of a survey

Anyone who has attempted a study using ordinary clinical case notes knows the problems of unstandardised recording and missing information. For most epidemiological studies it is essential to have purpose designed records.

Record design

The aims of the design are to help standardisation, speed, and accuracy in recording under field conditions, and coding and retrieval of results afterwards. Writing takes time, and, where possible, non-numerical information should be ringed or ticked rather than written out. The layout should facilitate subsequent numerical coding and data extraction, with one answer box for each item of information. Copying takes time and may introduce errors; if the record can be precoded, results may go straight to the analysis. An orderly and uncluttered layout makes for fewer mistakes, in both the field and the analysis: results should be vertically aligned on the right of the page, well separate from questions and instructions.

The record starts with the subject's serial number in the study, followed by sufficient personal identification to permit any planned follow up (address for postal contact, full name, date of birth, and—if available—NHS number for later tracing of morbidity through general practitioners, or mortality through the NHS Central Registry). If general practitioner or hospital follow up is envisaged, the subject's consent should be recorded on the initial record.

Records should be pretested, both in the field on representative subjects and in the office for subsequent coding and data extraction. It is impossible to foresee all the practical snags. In large studies the record design should be discussed with the statistician who will later be concerned in the analysis.

Questionnaires

The contrasts of clinical and epidemiological methods are epitomised by the approach to history taking. Clinically it calls for the highest skill—in establishing rapport with the patient, choice of questions, and distinguishing vague from convincing answers. In epidemiology, unfortunately, all unstandardisable skills must be excluded if comparisons are to be valid. Nevertheless, a good questionnaire is not so inferior to a clinical interview as might be imagined, for it concentrates on those few items which are most discriminating and eliminates what is superfluous; and for these key items the questions are phrased with maximum conciseness and clarity.

Closed ended questions, with one box for each possible answer (including "don't know"), are more readily answered and classified. Two short questions, each covering one point, are better than one longer question which covers two points at once. Questions which seem clear to a doctor may be difficult or understood differently by the subject, and pretesting is essential. Interviewers must keep strictly to the questions as printed and avoid supplementary questions if possible. Observer variation may often be avoided altogether by using self administered questionnaires.

Staff and training

In a small study the doctor himself may do all the work, but in large surveys he will need helpers. If an epidemiological examination technique requires skill and clinical judgment, it has probably been insufficiently standardised: if it is adequately standardised, it can usually be taught to any intelligent person.

The figure shows how two observers had distinct but opposite time trends in their performances during the early stages of a survey of skinfold thickness. Such training effects, which are common, should have been completed before the start of the main

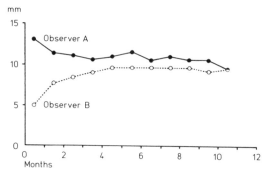

Trend in mean values for triceps skinfold thickness obtained by two observers in the same survey.

study: new staff need supervised practice under realistic field conditions followed by presurvey testing.

Despite all precautions, observer differences may persist. Observers should therefore be allocated to subjects in a more or less random way: if, for example, one person examined most of the men, and another most of the women, then observer differences would be confounded with true sex differences. To maintain quality control throughout the survey each examiner's identity should be entered on the record, and results for different examiners may then be compared.

Recruitment of subjects

At the MRC Epidemiology Unit in South Wales (a pattern setter in conducting surveys) a response rate below 95% is regarded as poor. Most people are willing to take part in medical surveys provided that they trust the investigator, just as patients will nearly always help their own doctor in his research. In population studies, however, there has usually been no previous contact. The selected subjects need an explanation of the purpose of the study, of why they in particular have been asked to take part, of what is expected from them, and what if anything they will get out of it (for instance, a medical check up, or a report on the research findings). Local general practitioners, too, need to know what is going on. Time given to public relations preparations is always well spent.

Response must be made as easy as possible. If attendance at a centre is required, it is better to send everyone an appointment than to expect them to reply to a letter asking whether they are willing to attend. Transport may sometimes be needed. Often the difference between a mediocre response and a good one is tactful persistence, including second invitations (by recorded delivery), telephone calls, identifying the reasons for non-attendance, and home visits.

Response rates

What response rate is acceptable? For an uncommon condition a response rate of 85% might be unacceptable, because a handful of cases in the unexamined 15% might greatly alter the findings; on the other hand, in a survey of smoking habits this response might be considered good.

In addition to prevalence, the acceptable level of response depends on the amount of bias. Non-respondents, and late respondents, tend to differ from those who come at first invitation. Those who did not reply to the first British doctors' smoking study subsequently had a mortality rate of 40% higher than those who returned their questionnaires. It is helpful to have some measure of the amount of such bias. Two approaches are possible. Firstly, a small random sample is drawn from the non-respondents, and particularly vigorous efforts are then made to encourage their participation, including home visits; the findings will indicate the extent of bias among non-respondents as a whole. Secondly, some information must be available for all persons listed in the study population; from this it will be possible to contrast respondents and non-respondents with respect to basic characteristics such as age, sex, and residence.

Analysing results

Epidemiological surveys quickly amass a lot of data. A study of 500 persons could easily yield 50 000 items of information, and for large studies there would nowadays be no alternative to computer analysis. Modern microcomputers have enough power to analyse small to medium sized studies if appropriate software is available. Library programs are widely available for the input and analysis of survey results, and in academic centres there will be no problems; for service computer units, however, there may be difficulties in obtaining and manipulating unfamiliar programs. The first essential always is for the user to know exactly what he needs. Some familiarity with survey analysis will help him to request tabulations which are simple to obtain rather than those which demand much special programming.

Many small surveys can be adequately analysed by manual tabulation of results and a desk calculator. The investigator gets the real "feel" of the data, which in a computer are instantly lost to sight. Moreover, programmable calculators take much of the tedium out of statistical calculations. Unfortunately, the data have to be read in afresh for each calculation, and if multiple analyses are needed a computer is still the method of choice.

Comparing rates

"Is this disease increasing? Does it occur with undue frequency in my local community? Does its incidence correlate with some hypothesised cause? Has the outcome changed since control measures were instituted?" To answer such questions means setting two sets of rates side by side and making some sense of the comparison. This section will examine some of the problems which may arise.

Terminology and classification of diseases

Diagnostic labels and groupings are many and various, and in continual flux: in the interests of communication some standardisation is necessary, even though no single system can meet all requirements.

The ICD system

The *International Classification of Diseases, Injuries, and Causes of Death*, published by the World Health Organisation, assigns a 3 digit numerical code to every major condition. Often a fourth digit is added for more exact specification: for example, ICD 205 is "myeloid leukaemia", which may additionally be specified as 205.0 "acute" or 205.1 "chronic". Broader groupings are readily formed—for example, ICD 200–208 consists of all neoplasms of lymphatic and haematopoietic tissue. This system is used for coding death certificates. It determines the presentation of results in the Registrar General's reports, and in the diagnostic registers of most hospitals.

Periodically, the system has to be revised to keep pace with medical usage. The new (9th) revision came into general use in 1979—consequently, some rates published before and after this year are not directly comparable.

In interpreting time trends it is also essential to consider changes in diagnostic standards and clinical terminology. Historical epidemiology is a dangerous pursuit, but errors are less likely if the analysis deals in broad disease categories. For example, coronary heart disease mortality rates in American men declined between 1968 and 1974 by 22%. One explanation for this might be that deaths formerly attributed to this cause are now being called something else (hypertension, cardiomyopathy, or viral myocarditis). The case for a real decline is much strengthened by finding that the trend applies also to "all cardiovascular diseases", and even to total (all causes) mortality.

Confounding variables

In an ideal laboratory experiment the investigator alters only one variable at a time, so that any effect he observes can only be due to that variable: all associations are either causal or due to chance. Most epidemiological studies are observational, not experimental, and compare people who differ in all kinds of ways, known and unknown. Analytic epidemiology is concerned with the attempt to isolate the effect of one key factor from among a tangled mass of confounding variables, any of which might explain the observed result.

According to the Hospital Inpatient Inquiry the case fatality ratio for acute coronary heart disease is higher in women (27%) than in men (21%). This is a statement of fact: the problem comes in its interpretation. Does female sex as such adversely affect prognosis, or is the result due to some confounding variable such as age? Simple cross classification (table I) produces a surprising result. The crude (all ages) rate is higher in women, and yet no real difference is seen within any individual age class. Age powerfully influences fatality, whereas sex as such has no effect at all; the crude rate is misleading simply because a higher proportion of the women patients come from the older, higher risk ages. This leads to a basic rule of epidemiological analysis: *"Crude rates must never be used to compare populations of different structure"*.

TABLE I—*Case fatality for acute coronary heart disease in hospital admissions*

Age (years)	Case fatality ratio (%) (and No of patients)	
	Men	Women
15–44	5 (6300)	3 (1200)
45–64	13 (45 600)	14 (13 700)
≥65	36 (31 800)	35 (27 700)
Total	21	27

Crude rates are not false but they are often misleading, because they fail to take into account other variables, particularly age. Every epidemiological report should describe the age structure of its study group and take account of it in the analysis. Cross tabulation is the simplest solution, and yields *age specific rates*.

In England and Wales the age specific all causes mortality rate for men aged 65–74 has not changed appreciably in the past 30 years, despite the great amount of medication that they now consume. This is a valid comparison of rates, even though there have been big changes in the age structure of the whole population and in the proportion of the elderly.

The method of cross classification and class specific rates is theoretically able to cope with multiple variables. In a study of bronchitis, for example, the prevalence (%) of persistent cough and phlegm could be cross tabulated by sex, age, and number of cigarettes smoked:

Age (years)	Sex	No of cigarettes/day			
		0	<20	20	>20
35–44	M	1·3	3·7	6·6	17·5
	F	1·5	2·9	7·0	15·7
45–54	M	..	..	..	..
..	..	..	..	..	..
..	..	..	..	..	..

The limitations to this approach are the indigestibility of large tables and a lack of numbers: most surveys are too small to examine all the interesting subgroups.

Standardised rates

In place of a cumbersome array of class specific rates one would often prefer the convenience of a single number to summarise the position after taking account of age and other factors. *Standardised* or *adjusted rates* provide for this need. Two techniques are available.

Direct standardisation

In the USA over the past 10 years deaths from coronary heart disease are said to have been declining in all age groups. How can the overall trend be summarised? Crude rates cannot be used, because the population's age structure has changed. Direct standardisation includes a *weighted average* of the age specific rates in each year, with weights equal to the proportion of persons in each age group in a convenient reference population (for example, the whole nation in the mid-point of the period). For men in 1968 the procedure is as shown in table II. Table III shows the standardised rates for men and women in the ensuing years, calculated in the same way. They show a remarkable fall.

TABLE II—*Example of direct standardisation*

Age (years)	CHD deaths/100 000 (1)	% of reference population in age group (2)	(1) × (2)
35–44	93	34·4	3 199·2
45–54	355	36·0	12 780·0
55–64	961	29·5	28 349·5
Total		100	44 328·7 ÷ 100 = 443

Indirect standardisation

The direct method is for large studies, and in most surveys the indirect method yields more stable risk estimates. Suppose that a general practitioner wants to test his impression of a local excess of chronic bronchitis. Using a standard questionnaire, he examines a sample of middle aged men from his list, and finds that 45 have

TABLE III—*Coronary heart disease in USA (ages 35–64): changes in age standardised mortality rates (deaths/100 000/year)*

	1968	1969	1970	1971	1972	1973	1974
Men	443	430	420	413	408	399	377
Women	134	126	126	124	120	118	111

TABLE IV—*Example of indirect standardisation*

Age (years)	No in study (1)	Symptom prevalence in reference group (2)	Expected cases = (1) × (2)
35–44	150	8%	12
45–54	100	9%	9
55–64	90	10%	9
Total			30

persistent cough and phlegm. Is this excessive? His calculation is shown in table IV.

First he sets out the number of subjects in each age class (column 1). He must then choose a suitable reference population in which the class specific rates are known (column 2). (In mortality studies this would usually be the nation or some subset of it, such as a particular region or social class; in multicentre studies it could be the pooled data from all centres.) Cross multiplying columns 1 and 2 for each class gives the expected *number* of cases in a group of that age and size, based on the reference population's rates. Summation over all classes yields the total expected frequency, given the size and age structure of that particular study. Where 30 cases were expected he has observed 45, giving an age adjusted *relative risk* or *standardised prevalence ratio* of 45/30 = 150%.

A comparable statistic, the *standardised mortality ratio* (SMR) is widely used by the Registrar General in summarising time trends and occupational differences. Thus in 1971 the SMR for death by accidents in doctors was 180%, indicating a large excess relative to the population at the time. To analyse time trends, as with the cost of living index, an arbitrary base year is taken.

Other standardisation techniques

Life expectation is an age adjusted summary of current all causes

35

mortality, being the average number of years that an individual would expect to live if exposed to the current age specific rates. More tedious to calculate than an SMR, its meaning is more evident. Thus the current life expectation for men in the north west region of England and Wales is only 67·9 years, compared with 71·3 years in East Anglia.

Regression techniques are an efficient means of standardisation and, thanks to computers, they are increasingly popular. The regression line relating ventilatory function to age, for example, may be used in a survey to correct each man's value to what would be expected at, say, age 40. Subsequent analysis employs these age corrected values. In *multivariate analysis* a computer, using regression or similar methods, can standardise for many variables simultaneously. Powerful though they are, these new techniques have by no means displaced the simpler and more robust methods of cross tabulation.

Prognosis and outcome

Inadequate knowledge of the prognosis and outcome of many diseases is a continual handicap in day to day practice. Decisions on whether to treat a patient with mild hypertension, whether to recommend an elective cholecystectomy in a patient with gall stones, or what prognosis to give the relatives of a patient with depression, all too often require data that are not available.

By itself, clinical experience cannot provide an adequate guide to prognosis and outcome. The two principal reasons for this inadequacy of clinical information are biased case selection and incomplete follow up of patients.

Case selection

For many diseases the cases seen by any one doctor are highly unrepresentative of all cases in the community. They are brought to his attention by a variety of selective factors, one of which is severity. Surveys have shown that many patients with peptic ulcer do not consult a doctor. Among those who go to their general practitioner the usual course of the illness is benign, with eventual complete recovery. But in hospital practice peptic ulcer frequently presents as a life threatening emergency.

Variation in tolerance of symptoms and demands for treatment are further selective factors. Surveys have shown no association between prostatic hyperplasia and social class, but among patients attending hospital because of this disorder there is a disproportionate number from social classes 1 and 2. People with hypertension who are referred to outpatient clinics are a notably miscellaneous and unrepresentative group of all hypertensive patients.

There are numerous examples of case selection. In hospital practice, it may be compounded by dispersing cases with the same disease among different specialties. Patients with giant cell arteritis, for example, may be under the care of neurologists, ophthalmologists, general physicians, geriatricians, or rheumatologists. The personal experience of any one specialist must necessarily be an inadequate guide to prognosis.

Incomplete follow up

A neurologist's view of multiple sclerosis tends to be unduly gloomy. Patients in whom the disease remits without residual disability (a third) do not continue to attend his clinic. Those in whom the disease runs a less favourable course return again and again. The general practitioner's view of multiple sclerosis is incomplete because the disease is rare, and no one GP will have more than a few patients on his list.

Clinical experience on its own is therefore an inadequate guide to the outcome of disease in which progression is slow and outcome variable. To some extent, every doctor's view of prognosis is unique and personal. (And so too is his view of the various clinical manifestations of a disease, a fact that authoritative statements in some medical textbooks take little account of.)

Two ways in which clinical experience may be supplemented are by follow up studies and record linkage.

Follow up studies

In a follow up study the progress of a group of patients diagnosed over a defined period of time is systematically observed. In order that the outcome in these patients may be generalised to groups of patients elsewhere, it is important that their method of selection is precisely defined. The age and severity of illness in patients admitted to coronary care units, for example, differ appreciably between units, and it is difficult to compare the experience of one unit with another. One possible response to this problem is to set up registers whereby all cases of diagnosed myocardial infarction occurring in a defined population, whether admitted to hospital or not, are recorded in collaboration with all local practitioners.

Life table analysis of kidney graft survival according to matching for HLA tissue types

Months from transplanatation	Good match		Poor match	
	No in study at start of period	Surviving period %	No in study at start of period	Surviving period %
1	47	87	271	71
3	39	76	191	53
6	34	74	139	45
12	32	62	113	41
18	26	60	102	37

The methodology of follow up studies is well established. The aim must be to obtain follow up data on all patients, since those who prove difficult to trace—because they default from clinic attendance or change address—may include a disproportionate number with a good or bad outcome. Possible methods of follow up, in addition to letters and home visits, include death certificate searches by the Registrar General, use of National Health Service central records, general practice lists, and employment pension records.

For diseases which are often lethal the outcome of a study may be expressed as case fatality or survival rates. *Case fatality rates* (the proportion of episodes of illness which end fatally) express the short term outcome of disease, but must be interpreted with caution. The definition of an episode of illness is not a specific period of time. Often it refers to a period of medical care, as in a coronary care unit, and case fatality rates may therefore be altered merely by varying the length of stay in hospital. To measure outcome over longer periods, *survival rates* are used. These show the proportion of patients surviving over a specified time from the date of diagnosis or the start of treatment. Survival rates may be corrected to allow for deaths from causes other than the disease being studied. As an alternative to survival rates, *life table* analyses may be used. An example is shown in the table. These analyses are more revealing than survival rates over one specified period, and are being used increasingly.

Record linkage

If the various patient records which are routinely compiled were to be linked together this would give a fuller picture of the course of an illness, and of different illnesses occurring in the life of an individual. One simple development of record linkage is matching hospital discharge and mortality data. Much needed information on life expectation after lethal disorders such as myocardial infarction at once becomes available.

There are many potential benefits in more complex linkages, for example between industrial employment and subsequent general practitioner and hospital consultations, but, because of the resources required and the problems of confidentiality, it seems unlikely that there will be much extension of record linkage in the foreseeable future.

The precursor and preclinical phases

Much current medical practice is concerned with patients in the late stages of chronic and incurable disease. A natural response to this is to identify these illnesses before they become clinically apparent, in the hope of identifying preventable or treatable antecedents. A simple but useful model of a chronic disease divides its evolution into three phases. In the precursor phase abnormalities—for example, a raised serum cholesterol concentration—are present without recognisable disease; in the preclinical phase the disease is established, but asymptomatic; in the clinical phase it is overt.

Identifying preclinical disease is the basis of screening and will be discussed in the next chapter. Among studies of the precursor phase the Framingham study is one of the best known. Some 5000 people aged 30 to 59 were examined annually over a 20 year period and initial concentrations of serum cholesterol and other measurements were correlated with subsequent morbidity and mortality. Among the important findings of this study have been recent observations on the inverse relation between ischaemic heart disease and concentrations of high density lipoprotein cholesterol.

There have been many similar studies. A recent one in Britain consisted of serial measurement of the forced expiratory volume (FEV 1·0) in 800 men over an eight year period. The lack of correlation between sputum production and the rate of decline of

FEV led to the concept of chronic bronchitis as two conditions—an obstructive and a hypersecretory disorder—which frequently coincide but are not causally identical. Studies such as these are an essential part of our attempts to arrest and prevent chronic disease.

Screening

Screening patients for preclinical disease is an established part of day to day medical practice. Routine recording of blood pressure, urine testing, and preoperative chest *x* ray films may all be regarded as screening activities; and the introduction of automated laboratory analyses has increased the scope of screening offered to patients in hospital and domiciliary practice.

Extending this activity to large scale services for people who have not requested medical aid has been the subject of much recent discussion and controversy. It places the doctor in a new role, whereby it is he who seeks out patients and recommends treatment rather than the patients consulting him. Doctors therefore have a special obligation to ensure that screening is beneficial. To this end, there are three questions which must be answered and for which epidemiological data are required.

Does earlier treatment improve the prognosis?

People with asymptomatic diabetes have a reduced life expectation. Nevertheless, two randomised controlled trials have failed to show that the prognosis is improved by treatment. In the Bedford study mortality after 10 years in a group of patients treated with tolbutamide was similar to that in a group treated with a placebo. In an American trial the cardiovascular mortality rate after eight years' follow up was reported as higher in patients treated with tolbutamide or phenformin, although some doubts have recently been raised about these findings. There is, therefore, no indication that large scale screening for asymptomatic diabetes is merited. This example illustrates that the outcome of screening must be judged in terms of its effect on mortality or illness, and not in terms of restoration of biochemical or other test results to normal.

In an American trial of breast cancer screening women were randomly allocated to a study group, which was offered annual screening, and a control group, which was not. Among the results was that the five year survival rate of breast cancer cases detected by screening was 83% compared with 58% among cases in the control group. Such a comparison can be made only if there is allowance for the fact that earlier diagnosis will, of itself, increase the interval between diagnosis and death and thus improve survival rates over a short period. The figures quoted are so adjusted, and allow for the so called "lead time"—the interval between the early diagnosis achieved by screening and the time when the disease would have been diagnosed without screening.

A further difficulty in this comparison of survival is that annual screening tends to identify cases of long duration, with a benign course, rather than cases where evolution is swift and fatal within a short period. This bias, however, does not apply to the main result of the study, which showed a reduction in the total number of deaths from breast cancer among the group offered screening as compared to the control group.

One facet of the effectiveness of treatment of asymptomatic disease is the definition of cases to be treated. In a previous chapter we showed that, since variables such as blood pressure have a continuous distribution within populations, there are no ready criteria for distinguishing "a case" from a normal person. Mild forms of the disease greatly outnumber severe forms. Somewhere towards the upper end of the blood pressure distribution there is a level above which treatment of asymptomatic cases will lead to a reduction in the frequency of strokes, heart failure, and renal damage. This level has yet to be defined precisely, and may vary from one population to another, but, for the purpose of screening, a case must be defined in terms of an operational level in so far as it can be determined from all the evidence—particularly that from clinical trials.

How valid and repeatable is the screening test?

Because a screening test must be inexpensive and easy to

perform, it is not usually the best diagnostic method for a disease. In screening, therefore, it has to be accepted that some cases will remain undetected. The *validity* of a screening test is measured by comparing its performance with a reference test, and table I shows the outcome of such a comparison. Validity is compounded of *sensitivity*, derived from a $(a+c)$, and *specificity*, $d/(b+d)$, which were discussed in the chapter on repeatability and validity.

TABLE I—*A contingency table relating the results of screening and reference tests*

Screening test	Reference test	
	Positive	Negative
Positive	a	b
Negative	c	d

For variables such as blood pressure, whose distribution is continuous and unimodal, a rise of the threshold separating "normal" and "abnormal" people will increase specificity at the price of a reduction in sensitivity. The competing needs for high sensitivity and specificity must be balanced. A high sensitivity takes priority if a false negative error is serious, as in screening for choriocarcinoma in women with a history of hydatidiform mole. High specificity is necessary when false positive errors must be avoided—either because of the needless discomfort and anxiety to individuals, or because of resources required for further investigation.

In addition to its sensitivity and specificity, the performance of a test is measured by the *predictive value* of a positive or negative result. For a positive result this is given by $a/(a+b)$, which represents the likelihood of a person with a positive test having the disease. When a disease has a low prevalence the proportion of true negatives $(b+d)$ in the population in relation to true positives $(a+c)$ is greater than when prevalence is high; and the proportion of false positives (b) will be greater in relation to (a). The predictive value of a positive result must therefore fall as prevalence declines. Understanding this point is of practical importance, for new diagnostic tests are usually first tested in hospitals or clinics, where prevalence is high. Despite satisfactory levels of sensitivity and specificity these tests may be disappointing when applied to the general population, because the yield of false positives is too great. Table II shows results from a breast cancer screening programme, using palpation and mammography, where the sensitivity was 67% and the specificity 98%, yet the predictive value of a positive screening test was only 20%.

Assessing a screening test requires not only a comparison with a reference test but also measurement of the test's *repeatability*, which shows the extent to which a single screening measurement may be taken as a sufficient guide to action. Where subject variation, observer variation, or measurement errors are large, repeatability will be reduced and a single test result may be unacceptable.

TABLE II—*Results of a breast cancer screening programme using palpation and mammography*

Screening	Breast cancer		Total
	Present	Absent	
Positive	127	497	624
Negative	63	19 313	19 376
Total	190	19 810	20 000

Sensitivity = 67% (127/190); specificity = 98% (19 313/19 810); predictive value = 20% (127/624).

What are the yields of the screening service?

The yield of a screening service is measured by the number of cases identified whose prognosis is improved as a result of their early detection. This must be related to the total number of tests performed. Theoretically, the yields of screening may be improved by restricting it to high risk groups, as has been suggested in the screening of infants for developmental and other abnormalities. But identifying relatively small high risk groups among whom most cases will be found is rarely feasible.

Although antenatal screening of women is widely accepted and practised, other forms of screening have proved less acceptable. The use of cervical cytology has been high in upper social groups, but low in social classes IV and V—where the disease has a higher incidence. Much has still to be learnt about methods of improving the acceptability of population screening, both in terms of changing people's attitudes and of the screening techniques that may be employed. The use of postal questionnaires, for example, requires further exploration. They are a cheap and acceptable technique in screening for hypothyroidism in high risk groups.

Ultimately, the yields of a screening service have to be balanced against the costs, in terms of staff and facilities, for screening and making the confirmatory diagnoses. For breast cancer screening it has been found that identifying one case requires examining 170 women by palpation and mammography and taking nine biopsy specimens.

Aetiology—comparison between communities

Occasionally descriptive epidemiology gives an immediate indication of the aetiology of a disease. The discovery of the relation between childhood lymphoma in Africa and malaria is one example of this. But, more usually, aetiological hypotheses arise from other sources, and their critical investigation requires special kinds of epidemiological data.

Clearly, only certain kinds of causative influence are accessible to epidemiological investigations, and no disease is the result of one influence alone. The concern of epidemiology is not to unravel the many interactions that result in illness, but to identify those determinants that are susceptible to manipulation, and, thereby, prevent disease. Epidemiological evidence about causation is often circumstantial and incomplete, but it is a guide to action.

A well known hypothesis suggests that lack of dietary fibre is a cause of a group of diseases, the so called "diseases of civilisation", which include appendicitis, gall stones, diverticulosis, ischaemic heart disease, carcinoma of the large bowel, hiatus hernia, and varicose veins. Epidemiological evidence to support such a hypothesis can be of three kinds: (i) comparison of communities with different amounts of dietary fibre intake to show that there are corresponding variations in the incidence or prevalence of the diseases; (ii) comparison of individuals to show that dietary fibre intake correlates with the presence or absence of disease; (iii) so called intervention studies, in which the dietary fibre of a population is increased, and the incidence of disease is seen to decline in relation to comparison populations whose dietary fibre intake remains unchanged. The first of these three kinds of evidence will be considered in this chapter.

Geographical variations

Central to the dietary fibre hypothesis is the rarity with which the "diseases of civilisation" are encountered in clinical practice in Africa and elsewhere in the non-industrial world. For at least some of these diseases, for example, ischaemic heart disease, the weight of evidence strongly favours the deduction that the rarity with which they are seen in hospitals and clinics reflects a low incidence in the population. Nevertheless, the frequency with which diseases present to doctors is sometimes a poor guide to their true frequency in the community; and in interpreting geographical data of any kind it is necessary to take account of three influences which may give a misleading impression of variations in incidence and prevalence.

The number of cases of a disease recorded by hospitals, clinics, or in special surveys is partly determined by people's willingness and ability to seek medical attention. Varicose veins are seen not infrequently during village surveys in Africa, but people with this disorder are less likely to seek treatment than in Western cities. Patients with acute surgical emergencies, such as appendicitis, are more likely to die before they reach hospital. Differences between industrial and non-industrial countries in the *levels of ascertainment* of disease are, of course, considerable. Such differences persist on a smaller scale within industrial countries, where patients' attitudes and access to medical care differ between rural and urban areas and from one region to another. In Britain, where almost all cases of perforated appendix or fractured humerus receive medical attention, the ascertainment of disorders such as depression or hypertension may vary greatly between the Highlands of Scotland and the suburbs of London.

In studies of international variations in disease frequency there is usually no standardisation of the diagnostic criteria for a disease. This may be of little consequence for disorders such as gall stones—which are readily recognisable—but for ulcerative colitis (which is sometimes included with the "diseases of civilisation") there must be definite *variation in diagnostic practice* between countries where bacillary and amoebic dysentry are common and those where they are not.

Non-industrial countries have a greater proportion of children than industrialised countries—where survival into adult life is more usual. In Iraq, for example, half the population is under 15. This must be taken into account when reviewing data on diseases of the elderly, such as diverticulosis. The difficulties posed by variations in *population structure* may be accommodated by age-sex standardisation (see the chapter on rates). Unfortunately this is often neglected. Knowledge of the world distribution of gall stones comes mainly from numerous necropsy series which have been documented over the past century. In only a minority of the published reports are ages recorded, and quantitative comparison from one country to another is therefore impossible.

Time trends

In Western countries in the past century there has been an apparent steep rise in the frequency of the "diseases of civilisation". Interpretation of such so called secular trends in disease is liable to the same difficulties as geographical variations. As health services have improved, so too has the ascertainment of disease; diagnostic criteria and techniques have changed; and the proportion of elderly people in the population has risen. Whereas with geographical variations differences in ascertainment, diagnosis, and population structure are accessible to current inquiry, documentation of secular changes is more difficult, dependent as it is on observations made and often scantily recorded many years ago. Nevertheless, the reality—if not the true size—of secular trends may sometimes be established with reasonable certainty. Discussion of the rise of lung cancer incidence during this century has been an instructive example of this.

Migrants

Further support for a hypothesis based on apparent differences in disease frequency among communities may be drawn from studies of migrants. Japanese migrants to Hawaii have seven times more carcinoma of the colon than Japanese in Japan, which suggests a close dependence of the disease on environment and

49

points to the need for dietary comparisons between the two groups. Interpretation of observations on migrants, however, presents certain difficulties, for the migrants may be unrepresentative of the population they leave. Norwegian immigrants into the USA, for example, have a higher incidence of psychosis than people in Norway. Although this may indicate environmental influences in the USA which lead to psychotic illness, it may also be a result of selective emigration from Norway of people more susceptible to mental illness, or of the unusual stresses imposed on immigrants during their adjustment to a foreign culture.

If the reality of geographical and time trends of the "diseases of civilisation" is accepted—notwithstanding the difficulties inherent in the data—they can be correlated with dietary variations. This will provide only circumstantial and inconclusive evidence of a causative link. In general, epidemiological evidence on disease causation is not rigorous; but it may be strengthened by using more than one method of study. Our next chapter considers methods that depend on comparisons between subgroups within a population rather than between different populations.

Aetiology of disease—comparisons between individuals

To test hypotheses about suspected causes of disease two kinds of epidemiological observations may be made on groups of individuals rather than whole populations. Using as an example the suggested relations between lack of dietary fibre and gall stones, these two kinds of observation are: (1) comparison of a group of people with gall stones and a group without, to show whether dietary fibre intake is lower in the former; and (2) comparison of groups of people taking diets of different fibre content to show whether gall stones are more prevalent among those on low fibre diets.

The first kind of observation is made in a *case control* study, comparing "cases" and a group of people without the disease. The second is made in a *cohort* study, comparing people with different exposures to the suspected cause. The case control method is more widely used by doctors, since the starting point is a group of patients, rather than groups of "normal" people in the population.

Case control studies

The cases in a case control study may be drawn either from all patients with the disease attending a hospital or clinic, or from patients identified during some form of population survey. The latter source is preferable in that it will give a more representative group of cases (see "case selection", page 37). The choice of cases for the study will require a predetermined definition of what constitutes a case (page 5) and a decision on the source of cases. Incident, that is newly diagnosed, cases are usually preferred to prevalent, that is existing, cases. A disadvantage of using patients with longstanding disease is that their memory of exposure to a suspected cause before the onset of illness may be inaccurate. Occurrence of a disease may alter a patient's lifestyle and the consequences of a disease may therefore be confused with its causes. Prevalent cases represent the survivors from all incident cases and factors influencing survival may be mistaken for causes of the disease.

Possible sources of controls for case control studies include groups of patients with other diseases, the general population, neighbours, and relatives. The choice of a source is partly determined by the need for cases and controls to be matched in respect of confounding variables. The principles of matching are described in the next chapter. When controls are matched to cases on, for example, sex and three categories of age the six age–sex groups are referred to as *matching strata*.

Although the cases in case control studies are not usually selected from a precisely defined population, it is useful to consider that they belong to a hypothetical one, comprising all individuals who, if they developed the disease, would be included as cases but are otherwise potential controls. The controls for a study are chosen so that they are representative of the population in respect of exposure to the suspected cause, within each matching stratum.

As a general rule, when patients with other diseases are used as controls it is wise to choose a variety of diseases. A study of the link between cigarette smoking and bladder cancer was rightly criticised because all the controls were drawn from a respiratory clinic. The smoking habits of patients with respiratory disease are not representative of the population. This is an example of *selection bias*. In this instance the association between the "control" diseases and the suspected cause could have been foreseen, but other such associations may be unforeseeable and selecting controls from a variety of patient groups mitigates this difficulty.

Matched controls drawn from the general population usually represent the ideal in a case control study, but pose practical difficulties. Nevertheless, with the advent of patient registers general practitioners have a ready framework for sampling. Electoral rolls, school registers, employment registers, and other listings may also be used, depending on the problems being investigated. Whatever source is used, the manner of selection of individual controls should be defined and orderly—for example, consecutive consultations or a formally drawn sample—rather than based on convenience. Using "healthy volunteers" is likely to introduce bias and is rarely satisfactory. The use of neighbours or relatives as controls is determined by the need to match out certain kinds of variables (see next chapter).

During the study observations should be made on the controls in the same conditions as the patients. Unavoidably the latter, because they are ill, may give more considered replies to questions about influences such as diet that might have caused their illness. But if dietary histories are obtained from patients while they are in hospital and from controls in their own homes additional bias may be introduced. This would be an example of *ascertainment bias*.

The statistical methods of analysis of case control studies are complex and beyond the scope of this book. It is wise to seek expert guidance. The complexity arises from problems such as the need to take account of paired matching of cases and controls.

A finding that the dietary fibre intake of patients with gall stones was generally lower than that of the controls would suggest an association between the two. Interpretation of this requires that three questions be answered. Firstly, could this apparent association be the result of some bias in the investigation? Bias is rife in case control studies: selection and ascertainment bias are the two main forms. Secondly, is it likely that chance alone has produced the association? Significance tests may be used to help resolve this. Thirdly, if the association is real, is it most reasonably explained on the basis of cause and effect?

Cohort studies

In a cohort study two or more groups of people (the cohorts) are selected by reason of their differing exposure to the suspected cause—in this instance, dietary fibre. The outcome—the frequency of gall stones—must then be determined among them. The starting point of the study is not, therefore, a group of patients, and the practical difficulties of cohort studies are generally much greater than in case control studies. If a disease is an uncommon outcome of exposure then large cohorts will be necessary. If the latent period between exposure and disease is long, the study may have to continue for many years.

Fortunately, it is sometimes possible to carry out cohort studies without massive resources or a prolonged commitment. The method is widely used in studies of industrial hazards. Data on exposure to the hazards among a group of employees may be obtained retrospectively from factory records, and the occurrence of disease among the employees may be ascertained from subsequent hospital and mortality records.

Because cohort studies tend to be time consuming and costly, they are usually reserved for testing precisely formulated hypotheses. Generally case control studies are used for exploratory investigations, and it is a particular strength of the method that a single study can simultaneously explore several causal hypotheses.

Risk

Where a = the incidence of disease in those exposed, and b = the incidence in the non-exposed, the *relative risk* is a/b. It is a measure of the strength of a suspected cause. For example, smoking is associated with a doubling of cardiovascular mortality in hypertensives. In a cohort study it can be calculated directly. In a case control study it can only be estimated indirectly.

The *attributable risk* is calculated as (a–b) and represents the risk to an individual of developing the disease following exposure. It is a measure in absolute units of aetiological outcome. For example among hypertensives, the excess in cardiovascular deaths in smokers may amount to seven per 1000 patient years. The attributable risk, not the relative risk, should be the guide to management and policy decisions.

Both relative and attributable risks express the risk to individuals, not populations. To the population a rare risk (like ethmoid cancer in High Wycombe woodworkers) is unimportant, whereas a common risk (like smoking in hypertensives) is serious. The product of (individual) attributable risk and the prevalence of the exposure factors gives *the population attributable risk*, and it measures the health burden of the factor to the population and thus the potential benefit of controlling it.

A small risk to individuals tends to be ignored; but if many people are exposed to it, then the population burden can be large. In the table it is seen that in individual mothers under the age of 30 the risk of a Down's syndrome birth is tiny; but because there are so many of them, they collectively yield half the cases. This limits the success of control measures in high risk subgroups.

Individual and population risks of Down's syndrome according to maternal age.

Maternal age (yr)	Individual risk %	% of births in age group	% of Down's syndrome in age group
<30	0·07	78	51
30−	0·13	16	20
35−	0·37	5	16
40−	1·31	0·95	11
>45	3·46	0·05	2
All ages	0·51	100	100

Aetiology of disease—
selection of controls

In the last chapter we gave a brief account of the two kinds of epidemiological study, cohort and case control studies, which are used to test aetiological hypotheses. Crucial to these studies is the selection of appropriate controls—an exacting procedure that requires careful planning.

At the outset it must be noted that the word "control" is being used in a particular sense. A biochemist seeking to determine the normal range of values for a new blood test will require specimens from a group of "controls". Ideally, he would obtain specimens from a random sample of the population, and his difficulty is the practical one of ensuring that the actual group of people he uses as controls—for example, hospital patients—are not so unrepresentative of the population at large that measurements made on them will differ greatly from population values.

Cohort studies

In aetiological studies the difficulty is that the control groups required are not random samples of the population, because some form of matching of study and control groups is necessary. In cohort studies the principles of matching are readily identified. Consider, for example, a study of the association between oral contraceptives and deep vein thrombosis. Two groups of women, one using oral contraceptives (the study group) and one not doing so (the control group), are to be followed up over a period and the occurrence of thrombosis among them compared. This is analogous to a clinical trial except that the participants are not randomly allocated to the two groups, but are allocated by the many cultural and social influences that determine use of oral contraceptives. In so far as these factors influence and independently affect susceptibility to thromboembolic disease they will also affect the comparison between the two groups.

Clearly the investigator must attempt to select two groups of women who, in so far as knowledge of the disease permits, are equally susceptible to the disease. Therefore, in this example, the distributions of variables such as age and parity must be similar. Factors which are associated with exposure to a suspected cause of disease and, independently, with the disease are known as *confounding variables* and the two groups must be matched in respect of them. Alternatively, the effect of confounding variables may be allowed for during the analysis.

As mentioned in the last chapter the cohort method is widely used in studies of industrial hazards. In these studies national statistics may be a convenient source of control data, allowing, for example, calculation of the number of lung cancer deaths which would be "expected" if the particular workforce was subject to the average national rates. However, it is usually wise to calculate an additional "expected" number based on local rates, since the rates for many diseases vary markedly from place to place. A control group of other workers in same industry, with different levels or durations of exposure to a suspected hazard, may reveal a "dose response" relationship following exposure.

Case control studies

Despite the apparent practical simplicity of the method the theory of case control study design is complex. A particular difficulty lies in the selection of controls. Suppose a doctor is recording each new case of deep vein thrombosis among women and wishes to carry out a case control study, comparing the frequency of use of oral contraceptives among his patients with that in a control group who have not had thrombosis. A control group consisting of a random sample of women of childbearing age in the community would clearly be inappropriate. If more patients than controls used oral contraceptives there would be several possible explanations other than that contraceptives are causally related to thrombosis. There may be confounding variables, such as socioeconomic influences, that are associated with the occurrence of thrombosis and, independently, with the use of oral contraceptives. The cases and controls must therefore be matched for confounding variables—or allowance for them made during analysis—before any conclusions about causality can be made.

Confounding variables must be distinguished from two kinds of variable for which matching is not required. The investigator may identify variables which influence whether a woman uses oral contraceptives, but are unlikely to have an independent association with deep vein thrombosis. Religious belief is an example. Matching on variables associated with the suspected cause but not, independently, with development of the disease tends to conceal the association being investigated. In an extreme case matching on all such variables would result in the frequency of use of the contraceptive pill being identical in cases and controls. This is over matching.

The investigator may also identify variables which influence the likelihood of thrombosis but probably do not influence whether a women uses oral contraceptives. The presence of varicose veins is an example. Matching on such variables, associated with the disease but not, independently, with the suspected cause, is generally without effect.

Methods of matching

Matching may be carried out either in groups, so that the overall distribution of confounding variables is the same among the cases and controls, or individually, so that each case is paired with one or more controls from the same matching strata. Either way, some degree of protection against error is afforded by using several controls for each case.

In the previous chapter we wrote that matched controls from the general population usually represent the ideal in a case control study. Patients with diseases other than the one being studied are often convenient. Sometimes matching is most easily accomplished by using patients' relatives as controls. For example, it was found that the average IQ of children whose mothers were anaemic during pregnancy was below average, at 97.4. To investigate a possible connection between anaemia of pregnancy and brain impairment in the child, it was necessary to exclude confounding socioeconomic variables, because anaemia of pregnancy occurs more often in families where the general level of education and measured intelligence are low. Matching to exclude these socioeconomic variables was most readily achieved by using a control group consisting of the brothers and sisters of the children. The mean IQ of the children born after pregnancies complicated by anaemia was the same as that of their brothers and sisters born after uncomplicated pregnancies.

When confounding variables are geographically localised—for example, variables relating to quality of housing—matching cases and controls may be most readily accomplished by using neighbours as controls.

In practice, the number of potential controls is often limited and the constraints of rigorous matching criteria may lead to insufficient being available. Sometimes, if individual matching is restricted to the dominant confounding variables, it is possible to allow for other variables by group matching during the analysis. At other times, the investigator may have to accept that the number of confounding variables is such that the case control method is not feasible.

No matter how rigorously a case control study is carried out the method is such that confirmation of the findings will usually be required from repeat studies. Although some of the case control studies on smoking and lung cancer are open to criticism because of the method of selection of controls or cases, their results provided strong evidence of the association because they consistently showed higher smoking rates in the cases than controls, albeit the magnitude of the difference varied from study to study.

Experimental studies

Epidemiological studies of causation, such as we have outlined in preceding chapters, rarely incriminate a factor to the extent that immediate action to remove or control it in the environment is justified. The evidence linking lung cancer and cigarette smoking is exceptional in this respect. Among additional kinds of evidence which may be brought to bear are the results of some form of experiment in which a group of people is removed from exposure to the factor and their subsequent disease experience compared with that among people in whom exposure continues. Historically such experiments have provided compelling proof of causation, confirming, for example, the dietary origins of pellagra and the link between retrolental fibroplasia and oxygen treatment. Nevertheless, they are not necessarily appropriate models for studies which are required today. For the diseases of industrialisation, such as ischaemic heart disease, there is no evidence of a single major cause whose manipulation would drastically reduce incidence. Rather, there appears to be an array of interacting causes, and experimental verification of any one of them would mean studying thousands of people.

Mortality changes in Scunthorpe after introducing public water softening in 1958, compared with those in the neighbouring town of Grimsby, where water remained hard[1]

	Scunthorpe		Grimsby	
	1950–3	1964–7	1950–3	1964–7
Water hardness (ppm)	488	100	250	250
Cardiovascular deaths per 100 000 a year	568	704 (+24%)	634	549 (−13%)

[1]Robertson J S. *Lancet* 1968; ii: 348.

Experimental evidence of a kind may be obtained by critical assessment of unplanned experiments. The table shows the rise in ischaemic heart disease mortality after softening of the water supply to Scunthorpe. The change in mortality is compared with that in the neighbouring town of Grimsby, where the supply was unchanged and where mortality fell slightly. The limitation of this kind of evidence is that comparison with Grimsby may be biased by many influences that affect deaths from ischaemic heart disease in the two towns and for which adequate allowance cannot be made during analysis.

Hopes for preventing diseases of industrialisation rest more on modifying personal behaviour, in respect of such factors as diet, smoking, and exercise, than on large scale changes in the environment—such as control of atmospheric pollution—which have been effective in the past. In the absence of results from planned experiments, the benefits of changed behaviour may be assessed by comparing the experiences of people who elect to change with those who do not. Unfortunately, this self selection of the experimental group introduces biases which may nullify any results. To take an extreme example, certain groups of people who stopped smoking subsequently had a higher mortality from cardiorespiratory diseases than those who continued to smoke. Presumably this indicates that people may change their smoking habits because of incipient ill health, rather than that it is harmful to stop smoking.

Assessing preventive measures

Strong reasons exist why the assessment of possible preventive measures should not depend solely on unplanned and imperfectly controlled experiments. Whereas in the past the consequences of mistaken conclusions about the effectiveness of preventive measures might not have been serious, this may no longer be so. Hitherto, the available methods of prevention have generally been removal of some noxious influence such as water pollution. Today, prevention may require introducing substances—fluoride in the water supply, polyunsaturated fats in the diet, oral contraceptives—whose long-term hazards cannot be known with certainty. Where positive measures, such as whooping cough vaccination, were introduced in the past they were to combat diseases that were widespread and lethal. When the incidence of disease is lower the

61

hazards of a preventive measure give more concern, and recent reassessment of the justification for mass whooping cough vaccination reflects this. This reassessment was feasible only in relation to those complications of vaccination that are acute and generally obvious. Assessment of long term complications of vaccination, diet, or any preventive measure, poses formidable problems.

Despite the difficulties, large scale preventive trials must be carried out before introducing costly and possibly hazardous preventive services. Multifactor trials, in which people's behaviour is simultaneously modified in several different ways, are an approach to the prohibitive costs of mounting large scale trials of the contribution of any single factor to the aetiology of multifactorial diseases. In the UK Heart Disease Prevention Project, for example, the participants received screening and health education for a range of coronary risk factors. This trial did not measure the extent to which individual factors contributed to the aetiology but quantified the overall effect of the regimen and provided a pragmatic guide to further action.

Preventive trials

Preventive trials on populations are analogous to clinical trials on groups of patients, and the basic methods are therefore well known. Nevertheless, the practical problems differ. Selection of an experimental population, to be randomised into intervention and control groups, must be made in such a way that it is reasonably representative of the target population to which the measure, if successful, will be applied. Although feasibility will, in part, determine choice of the experimental population this cannot be the sole consideration. A doubt about the World Health Organisation trial on clofibrate arises because many of the subjects were blood donors, whose representativeness of the target population is questionable.

Preventive trials of measures such as health education campaigns may require random allocation of communities rather than individuals to the intervention and control groups. Thus in the Heart Disease Prevention Project participating factories were allocated to one or other group, receiving either a programme of screening for coronary risk factors and health education, or being left alone. As in clinical trials, once the two groups had been assembled it was necessary to ensure that by chance there were not important differences between them that might affect the incidence of the disease being studied. Thereafter it was necessary to ensure that the management of the two groups remained the same in respect of everything except the experimental measure.

There are numerous possible sources of bias in assessing the outcome of a trial—for example, it has been found that default from preventive trials is more likely in those who have not complied with the advice or treatment given. High follow up rates are one protection against bias, and achieving this for many participants (18 000 in the Heart Disease Prevention Project) is a formidable task.

A positive outcome of a trial, in terms of decreased mortality or morbidity in the experiment group, will require balancing of the magnitude of the decrease against the costs of mounting a definitive service for the target population. The statistical significance of a difference between the experimental and control groups will depend not only on the magnitude of the difference but on the number of participants. In a trial a statistically significant result may fall short of what is of practical importance. Conversely, and more frequently, a difference large enough to be of practical importance may fail to achieve statistical significance in a small trial. A trial may have a negative outcome either because the preventive measures are inherently ineffective or because compliance with them is poor. Either way, that particular preventive programme has failed—but it is important that there should be provision in the trial for measuring compliance so that potentially effective methods are not prematurely discarded.

Outbreaks of disease

Although communicable diseases have declined in industrialised societies, outbreaks of diseases such as influenza, gastroenteritis, and hepatitis are still important. During the 1957–8 influenza epidemic, for example, the death rate in England and Wales was 1 per 1000 population above the seasonal average; an estimated 12 million people developed the disease; and the work load of general practitioners increased fivefold. From time to time new communicable diseases such as Lassa fever, legionnaires' disease, and, most recently, the acquired immune deficiency syndrome (AIDS) appear in epidemic form.

Communicable disease outbreaks

In outbreaks of common communicable diseases such as gastroenteritis and hepatitis it is the clinician who must initiate the appropriate investigations. The routine for these investigations is also the model for studying non-infectious disease epidemics.

At the outset it is necessary to *verify the diagnosis*. Three patients with halothane induced hepatitis were referred to one university hospital. Investigation of an outbreak of infectious hepatitis was begun, presumably because the clustering of cases gave an impression of infectivity and unduly influenced the physician's diagnosis. With some diseases—Lassa fever, for example—urgency demands that immediate action is taken on the basis of a clinical diagnosis alone. But for most diseases there is less urgency and the clinician should remember that clusters of cases of uncommon non-infectious diseases sometimes occur, by chance or for some other reason, in one place within a short time.

From time to time errors in collecting, handling, or processing laboratory specimens may cause "pseudo epidemics". The Center for Disease Control in Atlanta has reported several such pseudo epidemics. In one, an apparent outbreak of typhoid occurred when specimen contamination produced blood cultures positive for *Salmonella typhi* in six patients.

If a disease is endemic (habitually present in a community) it is necessary to estimate its previous frequency and thereby *confirm an increase in incidence* above the normal endemic level. Pseudo epidemics may arise from sudden increases in doctors' or patients' awareness of a disease, or from changes in the organisation of a doctor's practice. When the endemic level has been defined from incidences over previous weeks, months, or years the rate of increase of incidence above this level may indicate whether the epidemic is contagious or has arisen from a point source. In the former there is a slow rise, whereas point source epidemics, such as occur when many people are exposed more or less simultaneously to a source of pathogenic organisms, arise abruptly.

To build up a description of an epidemic it will be necessary to take case histories to identify the *characteristics of the patients*. Patients who are notified or otherwise recorded are often only a proportion of those with the disease, and additional cases must be sought. Thereafter it is necessary to *define the population at risk*, and relate the cases to this. This will require mapping of the geographical extent of the epidemic.

Defining the population at risk enables the extent and severity of the epidemic to be expressed in terms of attack rates—which may be given either as crude rates, relating the numbers of cases to the total population, or as age-sex specific rates. It may be possible to identify an experience that is common to those affected by the disease but not shared by those not affected; and, from this, a hypothesis as to the source and spread of the epidemic may be formulated.

Modern epidemics

There are several examples of large scale epidemics due to chemical contaminants. Outbreaks of mercury poisoning, with resulting deaths and permanent neurological disability, have been reported from several non-industrial countries as a result of ingestion of flour and wheat seed treated with methyl and ethyl-mercury compounds. In Spain in 1981 20 000 people were affected by a new disease, named the "toxic allergic syndrome", the most striking feature of which was a pneumonitis. During the first four months of the epidemic more than 100 people died and 13 000 were treated in hospital. Epidemiological and clinical investigation showed that the cause was ingestion of olive oil adulterated with rapeseed oil.

Widespread environmental contamination is a new agent of epidemic disease. In 1973 a fire retardant chemical, polybrominated biphenyl, was inadvertently mixed with farm feed. The resulting contaminated meat and dairy products led to most of Michigan's nine million citizens having detectable concentrations of the chemical in their blood. The effects on their health are not yet known.

Increasing recognition of environmental hazards due to substances introduced by man into his environment, as a result of the application of new technology, has led to a demand for large scale monitoring systems based on automated record linkage. Whether or not such systems come into operation, clinicians' awareness of changes in disease frequency or of the appearance of clusters of unusual cases will continue to be crucial to the early detection of new epidemics. In this early detection of epidemics due to medication, clinicians have a special responsibility. The rise in mortality among asthmatics due to pressurised aerosols, and the occurrence of corneal damage, rashes, and various other adverse effects of practolol are two of many examples of epidemics resulting from prescription of new drugs.

New diseases

New diseases continue to appear. The name legionnaires' disease was given to an outbreak of pneumonia at a convention of American Legionnaires in Philadelphia in 1976. There were 29 deaths. This stimulated an intensive epidemiological investigation whose successful outcome was identification of a Gram negative bacillus as the causative agent.

From 1981 to 1983 some 2000 cases of the acquired immune deficiency syndrome (AIDS) were reported in the USA. The ratio of men to women was 15 to 1, and the epidemiology suggested an infectious agent usually transmitted by homosexual intercourse. AIDS seemed to be a new disease. Subsequent studies, however, showed it to be endemic in central Africa, but with a sex ratio of around 1 to 1 suggesting spread by heterosexual contact. Investigations of this kind are an exciting and dramatic application of epidemiology.

Further reading

Armitage P. *Statistical methods in medical research*. Oxford: Blackwell, 1971. A full and explicit reference work on statistics.

Barker D J P. *Practical epidemiology*. 3rd ed. Edinburgh: Churchill Livingstone, 1982. A short, practical manual of epidemiology for use in developing countries.

Lilienfeld A M, Lilienfeld D E. *Foundations of epidemiology*. 2nd ed. New York: Oxford University Press, 1980. A stimulating book on principles, with examples.

McMahon B, Pugh T F. *Epidemiology. Principles and methods*. Boston: Little, Brown, 1970. An authoritative and comprehensive book on epidemiological methods, mainly for postgraduates.

Morris J N. *Uses of epidemiology*. 3rd ed. Edinburgh: Churchill Livingstone, 1976. Full of forceful examples, this book has enlarged many doctors' understanding of how epidemiology can contribute to medicine.

Swinscow T D V. *Statistics at square one*. 8th ed. London: British Medical Association, 1983. Medical statistics made as simple as possible.

Witts L J. *Medical surveys and clinical trials*. London and New York: Oxford University Press, 1964. An interesting and practical book on the conduct of surveys and trials.

Index